PALEO DIET

30 Fast and Easy
Paleo Diet Recipes
Targeting Losing Fat
and Getting Fit for
Beginners to Athletes

Contents

Introduction

The Paleo Diet is one of the most popular diets around. And why not? It provides great health benefits - including weight loss - with delicious food! And you don't have to starve yourself with this one.

But many people are still not comfortable with giving it a shot thinking the allowed foods are "exotic," tastes like crap, or are hard to prepare. If you're one of them, this book is good news. In this book, you'll find 30 delicious and un-complicated Paleo Diet recipes that can help you hit the Paleo ground running. And more importantly, these recipes will help you see that not only is the Paleo diet a practical one but also a very tasty one.

So if you're ready, turn the page and let's begin!

Chapter 1: Paleo-Approved Foods

While you'll learn 30 different Paleo diet compliant recipes in this book, I want you to walk away with so much more than just the ability to prepare these 30 recipes but to be able to create your own recipes off the fly. You can do that if you know the foods that are Paleo compliant. These 30 recipes are like memorizing 30 different answers to 30 different algebra problems and knowing the allowed and disallowed foods is like knowing the formulas or general solutions, which will allow you to solve just about any algebraic problem. In this chapter, we'll start with the Paleo allowed foods.

Meats

- Beef
- Chicken
- Lamb
- Pork
- Turkey

Seafood:

- Haddock
- Salmon
- Shellfish
- Shrimp

- Trout
- Wild Caught Tuna (when possible)

Eggs (Preferably Omega3 Enriched or FreeRange Eggs)

Vegetables

- Broccoli
- Carrots
- Kale
- Onions
- Peppers
- Tomatoes

Fruits

- Apples
- Avocados
- Bananas
- Blueberries
- Oranges
- Pears
- Strawberries

Tubers

- Regular Potatoes
- Sweet Potatoes
- Turnips
- Yams

Seeds and Nuts

- Almonds
- Hazelnuts
- Macadamia Nuts
- Pumpkin Seeds

- Sunflower Seeds
- Walnuts

Spices and Salts

- Garlic
- Himalayan And Sea Salts
- Rosemary
- Turmeric

Healthy Fats

- Avocado Oil
- Coconut Oil
- Lard
- Olive Oil
- Tallow

Liquids

- Plain Water
- Green Tea
- Pure Black Coffee

Chapter 2: Paleo-Disapproved Foods

Just as important when it comes to eating Paleo are the foods you're not supposed to eat for successful fat loss, more energy and better health. A key principle that should make it much easier for you to determine whether or not you should be consuming a specific type of food item is this: avoid processed foods. If it doesn't look anywhere near its original form, that's processed and therefore, avoid it.

Grains

- Barley
- Rice
- Rye
- Spelt
- Wheat

High Fructose Corn Syrup and Sugar

Highly Processed Foods

- Foods Labeled As "Nonfat," "Low-fat," "Diet," Or "Sugar Free"
- Synthetic Meal Replacement Shakes

Legumes

- Beans
- Lentils

Dairy Products, Especially Low Fat Versions

Trans Fats, i.e., Hydrogenated or Partially Hydrogenated

Vegetable Based Oils

- Corn
- Cottonseed
- Grape Seed
- Safflower
- Soybean Oils
- Sunflower

Chapter 3: Paleo Breakfast Recipes

Now that you have a general idea of what foods are allowed and disallowed on the Paleo Diet let's hit the ground running with 30 deliciously healthy Paleo compliant recipes, starting with the most important meal of the day; breakfast.

1.Prehistoric Egg Muffins

Ingredients

- 12 pieces free-range organic eggs;
- 3 cloves garlic, chopped;
- 1/2 cup kale, chopped;
- 1/4 cup cilantro, chopped;
- 1/4 cup fresh basil, chopped;
- 1/4 cup green onion, chopped;
- 1/4 cup tomatoes, chopped;
- Pepper for tasting;
- Salt for tasting; and
- A bit of coconut oil for lining muffin molds.

Directions

1. Preheat your oven to 350 degrees Fahrenheit.
2. Line your muffin molds with coconut oil.
3. Beat the eggs thoroughly and add salt and pepper to taste.

4. Mix the chopped vegetables in and, after thoroughly combining, transfer the mixture into the oil-lined molds.
5. Place the molds in the oven and bake for up to 25 minutes.
6. Let the muffins cool outside the oven before taking out of the mold and enjoying.

2. Breakfast Omelet Ala Avocado

Ingredients

- 1 piece avocado;
- 2 tablespoons red onion, minced;
- 4 pieces eggs;
- 4 slices bacon;
- A dash of Tabasco Habanero hot sauce; and
- A tablespoon of fresh cilantro, minced.

Directions

1. Fry the bacon slices until you get your desired level of crispiness. When done, crumble them to bits.
2. Cut the avocado in 2 and scoop the flesh out of the pieces. Mash the flesh until you get your desired texture. Mix the onion and cilantro in the mashed avocado, followed by the bacon bits. Mix thoroughly.
3. Beat the eggs and make omelets from them. Fill the omelets with the avocado mashed mixture. Add some Habanero sauce if you want some spiciness and zing.

3. Morning Eggs Guacamole

Ingredients

- 1 piece medium sized hass avocado;
- 1 pinch of chili powder;
- 1 tablespoon fresh cilantro, chopped;
- 1 tablespoon jalapeno, minced;
- 1 tablespoon tomato, diced;
- 1 teaspoon red onion, minced;
- 3 teaspoons lime juice, fresh;
- 12 pieces large hardboiled eggs, peeled;
- Pepper for tasting; and
- Salt for tasting.

Directions

1. Cut the eggs in half in a horizontal manner. Scoop the yolks out.
2. Take 2 egg yolks and mash them well with the avocado. Discard the 10 other egg yolks. Mix the salt, pepper, cilantro, jalapeno, red onion and lime juice in and combine thoroughly.
3. Fold the tomato gently into the mixture.
4. With the mixture, fill out each of the halved eggs' hollows (where the yolks used to be).
5. Sprinkle with some chili powder - if desired - before enjoying.

4. Prehistoric Porridge

Ingredients

- 1 dash cloves;
- 1 dash nutmeg;
- 1 teaspoon powdered cinnamon;
- 1 teaspoon raw honey;

- 1/2 cup almonds, ground; and
- 3/4 cup coconut cream.

Directions

1. Melt your coconut cream over medium heat. Mix the almonds and sweetener in and stir cook for about 5 minutes.
2. Throw all the spices and the sweeteners in and adjust the spicy-sweet level by adding more sweeteners, if desired.

5. Paleo Scalleo-Cakes

Ingredients

- 2 pieces, whole eggs;
- 2 tablespoons coconut oil;
- 8 ounces cauliflower, chopped;
- 1 1/2 ounces of minced onions;
- 1 1/2 ounces of chopped scallions;
- 1/4 cup water; and
- 1/4 teaspoon, salt.

Directions

1. Cut the cauliflower florets coarsely. Mince them using a food processor or vegetable grater.
2. In 1/4 cup of boiling water, put all the minced cauliflowers, stir quickly, and cover the pan. Turn off the stove's heat and let the cauliflower steam for exactly 10 minutes.
3. When done, drain the water and remove all moisture from the steamed cauliflower florets through a fine mesh. Put them aside when finished.
4. Whisk 2 eggs in a separate bowl. Mix the chopped scallions, onions, and 1/4 teaspoon of salt into the beaten eggs and combine thoroughly.

5. Pour the mixture on a pan with 2 tablespoons of coconut oil over medium heat and fry for about 5 minutes. Spread the mixture evenly using a spatula. Flip the cake after 5 minutes or when golden brown and fry for 3 minutes more or until browned also.
6. Remove from the pan and enjoy!

6. Paleo Broccoli Cakes

Ingredients

- 1 handful fresh parsley;
- 1 pinch pepper;
- 1 small clove of garlic, diced roughly;
- 1 whole egg;
- 1/2 teaspoon baking powder;
- 1/2 teaspoon salt;
- 2 tablespoons green onion, chopped;
- 2 tablespoons pumpkin seeds;
- 3 tablespoons tapioca flour;
- 6 to 7 pieces medium sized broccoli florets; and
- Coconut oil for cooking.

Directions

1. Grind the broccoli, garlic, green onion, and pumpkin seeds into tiny crumbs using a food processor.
2. Throw the egg in and continue processing until everything's well mixed.
3. Throw the tapioca flour and baking powder in and process some more.
4. Heat the coconut oil in a pan placed over medium heat and in it, fry up to 2 tablespoons of the processed mixture for up to 3 minutes per side. Flatten the mixture slightly to create round cakes.
5. Do the same for all the remaining mixture.

Chapter 4: Paleo Lunch and Dinner Recipes

7. Paleo Pesto-Ghetti

Ingredients

- 1 ½ cup flat leaf parsley, without stems;
- 1 clove garlic;
- 1/3 cup of olive oil;
- 1/3 cup of unsalted and blanched almonds;
- 2 plum tomatoes, chopped;
- 3/4 pound of squash spaghetti noodles; and
- 3/4 teaspoon of salt.

Directions

1. To prepare the squash spaghetti noodles, pierce the squash with multiple holes and bake in a pre-heated oven from 45 minutes to up to 1 1/2 hours. You'll know that the squash is ready to be spiralized into spaghetti noodles when its outer skin turns soft.
2. Cut the squash in half when done, take out the seeds, and use a spiralizer or a fork to scrape out the flesh into noodles.
3. To prepare your pesto sauce, puree the garlic, salt, and parsley using a blender. Pour the olive oil in a thin flow while the blender continues to run. Then, throw in the almonds and pulse the blender to chop them well.

4. Boil salted water in a big pot and in it, cook the squash spaghetti noodles for up to 12 minutes. Drain the squash spaghetti noodles when done but keep 1/2 cup of the salted water in another container for use later on.
5. Toss the squash noodles with the pesto sauce, tomatoes, and the remaining salted water from earlier. Enjoy!

8. Paleo Chicken Lime

Ingredients

- 1 piece bell pepper, diced;
- 1 piece of onion, finely diced;
- 2 pounds chicken, with bones;
- 2 slices of dried lime;
- 2 teaspoons coriander powder;
- 2 teaspoons cumin;
- 2 teaspoons mild paprika;
- 2 teaspoons turmeric;
- 3 cloves garlic, pressed;
- 3 tablespoons of fresh lemon juice;
- 3/4 cup of cilantro;
- Black pepper; and
- Olive oil for drizzling.

Directions

1. Bring your oven to 350 degrees Fahrenheit.
2. In the meantime, break the lime into pieces and boil it in 1 cup of water. Let it set for up to 15 minutes. Prepare the onion, garlic, bell pepper, spices, and herbs while doing so.
3. After letting the lime set for 15 minutes, strain the pieces and cut them into even smaller chunks. Return the lime pieces back into the water in which

you boiled and set them and add the spices, bell pepper, lemon juice, herbs, onion, garlic, and another 3/4 cup of water. Ensure all are mixed very well.

4. Throw the chicken in and sprinkle some black pepper. Mix the chicken and all the other ingredients well before pouring everything into a baking dish.

5. Bake the chicken in the preheated oven for 1 hour. Mix the dish every 20 minutes or so. If the mixture becomes excessively dry, put some more water and mix it.

6. When the chicken's golden brown and tender, take it out of the oven. Enjoy with some olive oil drizzled onto it.

9. Paleoghetti

Ingredients

- 1 large onion, diced;
- 1 piece of bay leaf;
- 1 pound of beef (grass-fed), ground;
- 1 whole spaghetti squash, sliced in half and seeded;
- 1/4 cup of bacon, chopped;
- 2 cans of meaty tomatoes;
- 2 celery sticks, diced;
- 2 tablespoons of lard;
- 2 tablespoons tomato paste;
- 2 teaspoons dried oregano;
- 3 cloves of garlic, minced;
- 3 pieces carrots, diced;
- Parsley for garnishing;
- Pepper for tasting; and
- Salt for tasting.

Directions

1. In lard, cook your ground beef and bacon together. Set aside on a plate when done.
2. Over medium heat, sauté the celery, carrots, oregano, garlic, and onion in the same pan that you used to cook the bacon and ground beef until tender.
3. Throw the ground beef, bacon, tomatoes, tomato paste, and bay leaf in, taste if salt and pepper if desired, and let the Bolognese sauce simmer for about 45 minutes.
4. While the sauce is simmering, bring your oven to 350 degrees Fahrenheit.
5. While simmering the sauce and pre-heating your oven, cut your spaghetti squashes in half in a lengthwise manner. Take the seeds out. Place the halves on a baking sheet with the cut side facing down.
6. Bake in the preheated oven for up to 35 minutes. When done, remove from the oven and use a fork or a spiralizer to scrape the squash halves' flesh to create noodles.
7. Pour generous amounts of the cooked Bolognese sauce on the squash spaghetti noodles and garnish with parsley if desired.

10. Sautéed Mushroom Treat

Ingredients

- 1 head of broccoli rabe (rapini), trimmed stems;
- 1/2 onion, sliced into thin pieces;
- 1/2 tablespoon of coconut oil;
- 1/4 cup white wine;
- 2 cups shitake mushrooms, sliced;
- 4 cloves of garlic, chopped; and
- Salt for tasting.

Directions

1. Boil the rapini for 3 to 4 minutes to blanch it. Drain the rapini completely when done.
2. Sautee the onions in about a quarter tablespoon of coconut oil dashed with salt until browned and tender over medium high heat. Don't sauté for more than 6 minutes.
3. Throw in the garlic and cook for 3 more minutes.
4. Throw in the remaining coconut oil, mix the wine and shitake mushrooms in, and taste with salt. Bring the heat up to sauté further until you see the mushrooms become brown.
5. Throw the rapini in. Cover the pan and continue cooking until the rapini becomes tender. Then, simmer with cover for a few minutes more before removing from heat to enjoy.

11. Baked Carrotatoes

Ingredients

- 1 sweet potato, cut into half inch lengthwise pieces;
- 1 teaspoon of salt;
- 1/2 teaspoon pepper;
- 2 tablespoons dried thyme;
- 2 tablespoons olive oil; and
- 7 carrots, cut into half inch lengthwise pieces.

Directions

1. Bring your oven to 400 degrees Fahrenheit. While doing so, toss together in a large baking sheet the carrot pieces, sweet potato pieces, olive oil, salt, pepper, and dried herbs.
2. Place the tossed mixture in the already heated oven and bake for up to 40 minutes or just until both the carrots and sweet potato pieces are browned and

crisp. Keep watch every couple of minutes to ensure they don't overcook.

3. Once done, remove from the oven and allow to cool before eating or storing for later eating.

12. A Caveman's Chicken Pasta Lunch

Ingredients

- 1 pound chicken breast;
- 1 spaghetti squash;
- 1 teaspoon arrowroot powder to thicken recipe if needed;
- 1 teaspoon garlic powder;
- 1/2 cup sundried tomatoes, julienned;
- 1/2 lemon worth of zest and juice;
- 1/4 cup extra virgin olive oil;
- 1/4 cup pine nuts;
- 2 tablespoons coconut oil
- 3 ounces canned black olives, sliced;
- Basil;
- Pepper for tasting; and
- Salt for tasting.

Directions

1. Heat your oven to 375 degrees Fahrenheit. Prepare the ingredients while waiting for your oven to achieve desired heat.
2. Cut the spaghetti squash in half in a lengthwise manner and take the seeds out. In a baking sheet with 1/4 inch of water, place the squash halves with the cut sides facing down. Place the baking sheet containing the squash in the preheated oven and bake for up to 1 hour tops. You'll know the squash is good when the skin turns tender.

3. Take the baking sheet out of the oven and let the squash cool prior to scraping the flesh off the squash with a spiralizer or fork to create noodles.
4. Slice the chicken breasts into small pieces and sprinkle with pepper, salt, and garlic powder for seasoning. Sear the chicken breasts in coconut oil on medium-high heat for several minutes. Reduce the heat and allow the chicken pieces to simmer until cooked through.
5. Throw the sundried tomatoes, pine nuts, olives, lemon zest and juice, and arrow root powder in and mix with the chicken in the pan. Let the mixture simmer for up to 2 minutes more to let the mixture become thick.
6. Remove from heat, pour in the olive oil and combine well. Pour the mixture on the spaghetti squash noodles and garnish with basil if desired before enjoying.

13. China Chicken Treat

Ingredients

- 1 cup of chopped onions;
- 1 teaspoon of curry powder;
- 1 teaspoon of dried cilantro;
- 1 teaspoon of ground turmeric;
- 1/2 cup of sliced jalapenos;
- 2 cups of cut red pepper;
- 2 teaspoons of ginger root;
- 5 cups of shredded cabbage;
- 5 teaspoons of coconut oil;
- 6 cloves of garlic; and
- 8 ounces of skinless chicken breast fillets.

Directions

1. Cook your chicken, onions, jalapenos, and spices in some water until the chicken is completely cooked.
2. Put some more water and continue cooking for 3 more minutes.
3. In a separate pan with coconut oil, cook the cabbage and red peppers until they become soft.
4. Split the cabbage equally between two plates and top each plate with the cooked chicken to enjoy.

14. Paleotallian Eggs

Ingredients

- 1 1/2 cup of chopped kale;
- 1 teaspoon of Balsamic vinaigrette;
- 1/2 cup of cherry tomatoes;
- 1/2 teaspoon of coconut oil;
- 1/4 avocado;
- 1/4 teaspoon of minced rosemary; and
- 4 free-range eggs.

Directions

1. Melt the oil in a pan over medium heat. Mix 3 tablespoons of water in together with the kale, cherry tomatoes, and rosemary. Make sure all's coated with the oil so stir everything well. Cook up to 4 minutes with a lid. Stir once every minute and a half.
2. When you're done cooking the mixture, use a spatula to press down the tomatoes so that their wonderful juices can be released into the mixture.
3. Brush aside the cooked vegetable mixture and in the same pan, cook the eggs in together with a pinch of pepper. As the eggs are close to becoming cooked, fold in the vegetable (tomatoes and kale) mixture

you brushed aside and cook for up to 2 minutes more.
4. When you're finished, splash a teaspoon of balsamic vinaigrette over the cooked egg-tomato-kale and garnish with avocado to enjoy.

15. Prehistoric Burger

Ingredients

- 1 pound of ground grass-fed beef;
- 1 teaspoon of minced garlic;
- 2 tablespoons of almond meal;
- 2 teaspoons of basil;
- 3 sun dried tomatoes cut into very small bits.
- 5 eggs;

Directions

1. Combine the almond meal, basil, 1 egg, garlic, and sundried tomatoes well. From the resulting mixture, create 2 burger patties.
2. Cook the patties for up to 5 minutes per side or until you achieve your preferred level of doneness. As soon as they're cooked, place them on a plate.
3. Fry the remaining eggs one at a time and top the burger patties with them.

16. Paleo Pot Roast

Ingredients

- 1 1/2 tablespoons of cider vinegar;
- 1 medium-sized onion;
- 1/2 teaspoon of Allspice;
- 1/2 teaspoon of black pepper;
- 1/4 teaspoon of ground nutmeg;

- 2 bay leaves;
- 2 tablespoons of lard;
- 2/3 cup of beef broth;
- 3 tablespoons of lemon juice;
- 3 tablespoons of olive oil;
- 4 medium-sized tomatoes; and
- 4 pounds of grass-fed beef chuck.

Directions

1. Combine the allspice, nutmeg, and pepper very well. Rub the resulting mixture all over the roast on all sides. To help the roast absorb the mixture much better, use a fork to poke the roast with holes on all sides.
2. Core your tomatoes and once you're done, cut them into chunks. Put them in a blender.
3. Peel the onion and cut into small pieces. Place it in the blender together with the tomato chunks and pulse until everything's chopped.
4. Pour in the olive oil, lemon juice, and vinegar. Blend some more until the mixture achieves a thin consistency.
5. Put the roast in a Ziploc bag and pour the tomato-onion blended mixture in the bag. Zip the bag and put it in the fridge for at least 8 hours to marinate the roast.
6. After you've marinated the roast for at least 8 hours, sear both sides of the roast and melt the lard in a Dutch oven set on medium-high heat. Save the roast's marinade for later.
7. When the roast has been seared and the lard has melted, mix the reserved marinade, the beef broth, and the bay leaves in. As the mixture starts to boil, lower the heat so that it will come down to a simmer. Let the roast and the mixture continue simmering for 3 hours - with cover - or until you achieve your roast's preferred tenderness.

8. Take the roast out of the Dutch oven and transfer it onto a plate. Increase the heat of the Dutch oven again to help the juice inside it achieve a thick consistency, which you can use as a gravy or sauce to be poured over the roast before eating.

17. Stone Age Beef Shabu Shabu

Ingredients

- 1 large pot of bone broth;
- 1/2 pound of thinly sliced shabu-shabu beef;
- Spinach leaves; and
- Tamari sauce for serving, gluten free.

Directions

1. Boil the beef and the vegetables in the broth until you see the meat turn dark red or brown.
2. When done, enjoy with some tamari sauce.

18. Stone Age Sheep

Ingredients

- 1 cup of sulphite-free red wine;
- 1 pound of lamb steaks;
- 1 tablespoon of freshly cracked pepper;
- 1/4 cup of Balsamic vinegar;
- 2 fresh organic rosemary sprigs rosemary, leaves removed; and
- 3 tablespoons of extra virgin olive oil.

Directions

1. Wash the steaks. When done, put them inside a 3-inch deep dish.

2. Prepare the lamb steaks' marinade by mixing together very well all the remaining ingredients. Marinate the lamb in this mixture for up to 2 days.
3. After marinating, grill the steaks for up to 12 minutes on low heat per side or until your desired doneness level's been achieved. Baste the steaks with the marinade while grilling.

19. Drunk Chicken

Ingredients

- 1 clove garlic;
- 1 cup of organic Marsala wine;
- 1 sweet onion sliced thinly;
- 2 cups of rinsed and sliced Portobello mushrooms;
- 2 sprigs of fresh rosemary, stems removed;
- 2 tablespoons of red wine vinegar;
- 4 Free range organic chicken breast fillets;
- 4 tablespoons of extra virgin olive oil; and
- Freshly cracked pepper for tasting.

Directions

1. Bring the oven to 375 degrees Fahrenheit.
2. Put the chicken breasts inside a baking dish. Use the mushrooms to cover the breast fillets.
3. Combine the red wine, red wine vinegar, 3 tablespoons of extra-virgin olive oil, and rosemary.
4. Sautee the onion and garlic in 1 tablespoon of extra-virgin olive oil until tender. When cooked, spread over the mushrooms and chicken breast fillets in the baking dish.
5. Pour the red wine mixture on the chicken fillets and bake in the heated oven for up to 45 minutes or until your desired level of doneness is achieved.

20. Paleo Shrimpepper

Ingredients

- 1 1/2 pounds of peeled, raw shrimps;
- 1 tablespoon of coconut aminos;
- 1 tablespoon of fish sauce;
- 1 teaspoon of black pepper;
- 1/4 cup of fresh cilantro;
- 3 tablespoons of coconut oil; and
- 4 cloves of garlic.

Directions

1. Melt the coconut oil in low heat. Sautee the garlic in it for 3 minutes with frequent stirring. Don't let the garlic turn brown.
2. Throw the shrimps in and sauté until they turn pink or approximately 5 minutes. Mix the fish sauce, pepper, and coconut aminos in and continue sautéing for another 2 minutes.
3. Transfer the shrimps on a serving plate. Increase the heat under the pan to heat the liquid aminos further for up to 2 additional minutes.
4. Pour the liquids in the pan onto the shrimps and top with chopped cilantros to enjoy.

Chapter 5: Paleo Dessert Recipes

21. Stone Age Strawberry Ice Cream

Ingredients

- 1 cup of strawberries, frozen and chopped;
- 1 pinch of salt;
- 1 teaspoon of pure and natural vanilla extract;
- 1/2 heaping cup of sunflower seed butter;
- 2 cups of coconut milk (full fat);
- 2 pieces of egg yolk; and
- 3/4 cup of homemade strawberry sauce.

For The Homemade Strawberry Sauce:

- 1 teaspoon of lemon juice;
- 1/2 cup (packed) of dates; and
- 3 cups strawberries, frozen.

Directions

1. For the strawberry sauce, place the dates, strawberries, and lemon juice in a small pan placed over medium heat. Cook until the strawberries turn soft and its juices have been extracted. If the mixture starts to boil at any point, bring the heat down to stop the boiling.

2. Pour the mixture in a blender when done. Blend the mixture until everything turns into one smooth consistency mixture. Allow the mixture to cool before you pour it into a glass container for complete cooling inside the fridge.
3. Once cooled, blend the strawberry sauce, salt, coconut milk, vanilla, and the egg yolks until once again, you arrive at a very smooth consistency mixture.
4. Pour the blended mixture inside an ice cream making machine and churn according to the machine manufacturer's instructions.
5. When the churning is almost over and the ice cream has turned thick, mix in the chopped strawberries.
6. In a metal bowl over a pot of boiling water, place the sunflower seed butter to warm. Ensure the butter turns smooth before setting aside to cool at room temperature.
7. When the ice cream machine finishes churning, bring out the ice cream container. Pour a layer of the ice cream at the bottom of the container.
8. Drizzle the first layer with sunflower seed butter.
9. Pour another layer of the homemade ice cream in the container and drizzle again with sunflower seed butter. Repeat until all have been used up. Make sure the last layer is all ice cream.
10. Use a butter knife to mix the ice cream in the container before putting the container in the freezer for 2 hours.
11. Before enjoying, let the ice cream sit outside the freezer for 10 minutes before scooping away and devouring the treat.

22. Neanderthal Fruit Salad

Ingredients

- 1/2 cup of blackberries;
- 1/2 cup of blueberries;
- 1/2 cup of grapes, cut in half;
- 1/2 cup of kiwi, peeled and quartered;
- 1/2 cup of pineapples, sliced into ½ inch pieces;
- 1/2 cup of strawberries, quartered; and
- 1/2 cup of watermelon, diced.

Directions

1. Just mix everything! Then enjoy!

23. Banana Honey Fry

Ingredients

- 1 piece of banana, cut;
- 1 tablespoon of pure, raw honey;
- Cinnamon powder; and
- Coconut oil.

Directions

2. Lightly coat a skillet with coconut oil. Place it over medium heat and cook the banana pieces in it for up to 2 minutes per side.
3. Mix together 1 tablespoon of raw, pure honey and 1 tablespoon of water while the banana pieces are cooking. Make sure the mixture's whisked very well.
4. After you're done cooking the bananas, take the skillet away from heat and slather the banana pieces with the honey mixture.
5. Sprinkle with a little bit of cinnamon powder after the bananas have cooled down to enjoy.

24. Stone Age Choco Poms

Ingredients

- 1/2 cup of semisweet chocolate chips, melted; and
- 1 1/4 cup of pomegranate seeds.

Directions

1. Use liners to line a small muffin tin. Put 2 teaspoons of melted chocolate in each of the muffin tin's cups. Pepper the top of the choco-filled cups with pomegranate seeds before using more melted choco to drizzle each cup.
2. Place the muffin tin in the fridge for about 20 minutes or until firm.

25. Paleo Choco Berry Cubes

Ingredients

- 2 cups of chocolate chips;
- 2 tablespoons of coconut oil; and
- 16 pieces fresh strawberries, including stems.

Directions

1. Mix together well the coconut oil and melted choco chips in a medium-sized bowl.
2. At the bottom of each ice cube mold, layer a spoonful of the chocolate mixture.
3. Top each of the chocolate layered cube with a strawberry, with the stems protruding upward.
4. With the remaining melted chocolate mixture, fill up all the strawberry and chocolate filled molds.
5. Leave in the freezer for up to 5 hours to solidify the chocolate before enjoying.

Chapter 6: Paleo Snack Recipes

26. Popped Cauliflowers

Ingredients

- 1/2 head of cauliflower, diced small like popcorn;
- 1/2 teaspoon of dried chives;
- 1/2 teaspoon of onion powder;
- Extra virgin olive oil; and
- Salt.

Directions

1. Bring your oven to 450 degrees Fahrenheit.
2. In olive oil, toss the cauliflower pieces.
3. Drizzle salt over the olive oil-tossed cauliflower then spread on a parchment paper lined baking sheet.
4. Bake in the pre-heated oven for 30 minutes. In between, turn the cauliflower twice.
5. Remove from the oven and drizzle with chives and onion powder to enjoy.

27. Cantaloupe Prosciutto Wraps

Ingredients

- 1 tablespoon of fresh chopped mint leaves;
- 1/2 cantaloupe;

- 1/3 cup of balsamic vinegar;
- 2 teaspoons of extra virgin olive oil;
- 3 ounces of sliced prosciutto; and
- Fresh ground black pepper.

Directions

1. Cut the cantaloupe into 6 wedges before further cutting into 1.5-inch pieces. Remove the rinds.
2. Cut the prosciutto into strips that are 1 1/4 x 3 1/2 in size. Use the prosciutto strips to wrap each of the cantaloupe pieces, and use a toothpick to secure the wrap.
3. Prepare the balsamic glaze by heating the balsamic vinegar on a small-sized skillet placed over medium-high heat. Let the vinegar simmer for 3 to 4 minutes or just until you see the vinegar start to become thick and shrink in volume to about 1 tablespoon only.
4. Drizzle olive oil and the balsamic glaze on a serving plate. Put the wraps on the plate and drizzle with pepper and mint to enjoy.

28. Paleomus (Paleo Hummus)

Ingredients

- 1 head of cauliflower, cut into smaller florets;
- 4 tablespoons of tahini;
- 4 tablespoons of olive oil for the hummus;
- 1 tablespoon of olive oil for roasting the vegetables;
- 4 tablespoons of lemon juice;
- 1 teaspoon of salt;
- 1 teaspoon of garlic powder;
- 1/2 of a red pepper, sliced;
- 1/2 of an eggplant, sliced;
- 1/2 teaspoon of cumin;
- 1/4 teaspoon of black pepper;

- Paprika for garnish; and
- Olive oil for garnish.

Directions

1. Bring your oven to 400 degrees Fahrenheit.
2. Use aluminum foil to cover a cookie sheet. Pour a tablespoon of the olive oil on the cookie sheet and evenly spread it out over the sheet.
3. Place the cut up red peppers, eggplant, and cauliflower florets on the sheet and bake the vegetables in the oven for up to 40 minutes, flipping them at the midpoint of the bake.
4. When done, bring out the vegetables from the oven and let them cool.
5. Put the grilled vegetables, 4 tablespoons of olive oil, tahini, garlic powder, salt, lemon juice, pepper, and cumin in a blender and blend until you get a hummus-like texture.
6. Garnish the humus with olive oil and paprika when done.

29. Asparagus Prosciutto Wraps

Ingredients

- 1 bunch of asparagus;
- 1/4 pound of prosciutto;
- Pepper, to taste; and
- Optional olive oil.

Directions

1. Heat your oven to 350 degrees Fahrenheit.
2. Boil the asparagus in water for 2 minutes.
3. Immediately take the asparagus out of the boiling water after 2 minutes and put it in a bowl of water and ice.

4. After being cooled down, take 23 asparagus spears and wrap with prosciutto. Line them up on a baking sheet and drizzle with pepper and - if desired - olive oil.
5. Bake in the oven for 7 minutes or until crispy.

30. Sweet Rosemary Potatoes

Ingredients

- 1 teaspoon pepper;
- 1 teaspoon salt;
- 12 tablespoons olive oil;
- 2 medium size sweet potatoes, cut into 1" cubes; and
- 2 sprigs of fresh rosemary, chopped (or 1 tablespoon dried rosemary).

Directions

1. Heat your oven to 425 degrees Fahrenheit and place the rack in the upper third level. Use parchment paper to line a baking sheet.
2. Mix all the ingredients together in a medium-sized bowl and toss so that the sweet potatoes will be coated with the mixture.
3. Spread the coated sweet potatoes evenly on the baking sheet.
4. Roast in the oven for up to 30 minutes or until the potatoes turn golden brown.

Conclusion

Thanks for buying this book. I hope that more than just learning these 30 very delicious Paleo Diet recipes, you were encouraged to go to the kitchen and give these recipes a try a.s.a.p. These recipes won't mean much if you don't actually prepare and eat them. Only by preparing the dishes in this recipe book and others like it will you be able to experience the delicious health benefits of the Paleo Diet.

You don't have to prepare them all at once. Given there are 30 recipes here, try one recipe per day for one straight month. If it's too overwhelming, try 2 recipes weekly on different days. The important thing is you start cooking the recipes here and experience the Paleo Diet's delicious benefits.

Here's to your delicious health my friend! Cheers!

References

No sources used